WHY YOUR DOCTOR OFFERS NUTRITIONAL SUPPLEMENTS

REVISED SECOND EDITION

Stephanie Selene Anderson
with Mark R. Anderson

Design by Brian Gabel

Cover Art (front and back) Copyright © by Ginny Hogan
www.chilirosegallery.com
ginnyhogan@cybermesa.com

Photographs by Stephanie Selene Anderson

Second Printing

Note to the Reader: *The ideas and suggestions contained in this book are not intended as a substitute for the appropriate care by a licensed healthcare practitioner.*

Published by

Selene River Press

P.O. Box 270091
Fort Collins, Colorado 80527
866-407-9323
www.seleneriverpress.com
info@seleneriverpress.com

ISBN 0-9645709-1-2
PRINTED IN THE UNITED STATES OF AMERICA

Acknowledgments

With thanks to the sharp editorial services of Karen Grasso and Jane D. Albritton; the generous consulting services of the perspicacious Judith DeCava; and the hearty support of Kim Knight, Dean Turner, and Jane C. Mirandette.

We are grateful to the gracious Bonnie Antich and Scott LeCocq of Colorado for use of their Canyon Spirit Gallery and Bonnie's beautiful pottery.

Ginny Hogan's painting, "Spirit Hunters," captures the joy of the quest, and we are grateful to her for letting it speak from the covers of this book.

Instinct is extinct; but there are those who have kept knowledge extant.
–Mark R. Anderson

With everlasting thanks to Dr. Royal Lee

Table of Contents

The Quest For Superior Nutrition Has Never Been Easy

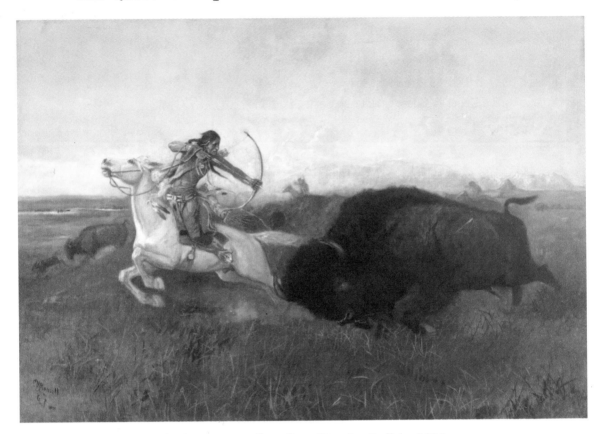

Charles M. Russell, *Indians Hunting Buffalo*, 1894.
Courtesy Sid Richardson Collection of Western Art, Fort Worth, Texas

Nutrition Derived from the Entire Buffalo

- Vitamin A from the kidney, liver, and fatty tissue. Nourishment for eyes, skin, lungs, kidneys, digestive tract, and immune system.

- Vitamin B complex from liver and muscle meats: including concentrated amounts of thiamin, riboflavin, niacinamide, folic acid, pyridoxine, pantothenic acid, B12. Essential sustenance for the health of the heart, nerves, brain, blood cells, fetal development, and energy creation.

- Vitamin C complex from the adrenals for strong bones, teeth, connective tissue (ligaments, tendons, cartilage, discs), and immune system function.

- Vitamin D from being outside and irradiating cholesterol in the skin with sunlight.

- Vitamin E from the organ meats supporting the heart, immune system, tissue repair, and endocrine system.

- Vitamin F from all the natural organ fats (including Omega 3, Omega 6, and essential polyunsaturated fatty acids) healthful saturated fats and cholesterol to protect cell membranes. This supported healthy heart, skin, hair, liver, gall bladder, endocrine glands, lymphatic circulation, respiratory tract, and brain.

- Vitamin K from liver for health of the blood and bones.

- Amino acids-rich protein from the muscle and organ meat. The meat provided all of the 8 essential amino acids plus a full spectrum of nonessential aminos. This protein also provided glucose for energy.

- Iron for the hemoglobin of the red blood cell from organ meats, especially liver. Essential for oxygen-rich blood.

- Nucleic acids (including RNA and DNA), Protomorphogens and cell determinants from organ meats and marrow. Essential nutrition for the brain and for organ/tissue repair.

- Enzymes for digestion and immune function and endocrine support from organs.

- Amino acids, collagen, calcium and minerals were obtained from bones made into soup stock yielding nutrient-rich gelatin. These nutrients contribute to strong connective tissues, like cartilage and ligaments, creating stable joints. The amino acids proline and glycine that are abundant in the gelatin have a strong connection to joint health. Gelatinous bone stock is a nutritious source of collagen, calcium, minerals and the amino acids. This is far superior to the gelatin common today which is made from animal skins. Soups made from bones are very healing to the GI tract by supplying hydrophilic colloids (a watery, gelatinous, glue-like substance that manages water content in the GI tract). Prior to metal pots, Plains Indians would use the stomach of the buffalo to slowly cook soups and stews high above an open fire.

- Minerals from organ meats and especially minerals from the soups made from bones including highly absorbable forms of calcium, phosphorus, magnesium, manganese, zinc, iron, copper, selenium, sodium, potassium and others. These minerals added important nutrient support to every system and tissue in the human body. The vast array of minerals from organ meats and soups gave constant support to these systems: nervous, skeletal, circulatory, endocrine, respiratory, skin, immune, and formed the basis for hundreds of essential enzymes produced by minerals in combination with amino acids.

...and the buffalo made all this out of grass and water.

Introducing

Why Your Doctor Offers Nutritional Supplements

Book I
in
The Quest for Superior Nutrition Series

Charles Russell's painting, *Indians Hunting Buffalo*, powerfully captures the sense of an uncertain outcome: Will this man and his family survive in health and strength, or will he and his horse lose their lives in the quest for superior nutrition? Such grave risk was commensurate with the reward of securing the best food possible for his family.

Before you become discouraged by having to re-direct your energies and routines in order to find sources of superior food, think of the American Indian who had to summon courage, artful skill, instinct, intelligence, and knowledge of the properties and characteristics of his food supply. Think of the need to risk life and limb to travel a minimum of hours, a maximum of months, from family and community to obtain the most superior nutrition.

Although we have ingeniously developed the means to free ourselves from the bodily risks and labors of this task, we have lost sight of the goal: superior nutrition. We must now achieve the mental equivalent of that physical labor. We have to exercise the same strength of will, awareness, care and knowledge, motivated by the same inherent quest: To obtain the most superior nutrition possible for our families.

The modern food supply falls far short of providing all that is necessary to produce robust, healthy people. We no longer live within a system that teaches children what foods and methods of preparation will provide superior nutrition. Consequently, many of us are trying to find a new way to educate ourselves and our families.

We have all tried turning to doctors for help, but often the doctor or health professional does not have the time or knowledge. Although there is no lack of written information on health and nutrition to turn to in lieu of professional help, without a confident awareness of the difference between counterfeit and original food, or a basic understanding of why the body does not thrive on counterfeit food, it is difficult to discern what information is accurate.

To assist you in this task, Selene River Press has begun The Quest for Superior Nutrition Series, and offers this first book, *Why Your Doctor Offers Nutritional Supplements*. This book provides, not a new fad diet, but a fundamental understanding of the link between our human health and the health of soil, plants and animals. *Why Your Doctor Offers Nutritional Supplements* also provides the doctor and health professional with a handy means of educating patients. Doctors and the general public alike will benefit from an honest look at The Seven Deadly Fallacies of the Western Diet, health food stores, and the inaccuracies of supplement information, all to help develop the discernment necessary to navigate oneself to the goal: Superior Nutrition.

The quest for superior nutrition has never been easy, but the reward is commensurate with the effort.

THE SUN: Source of All Energy

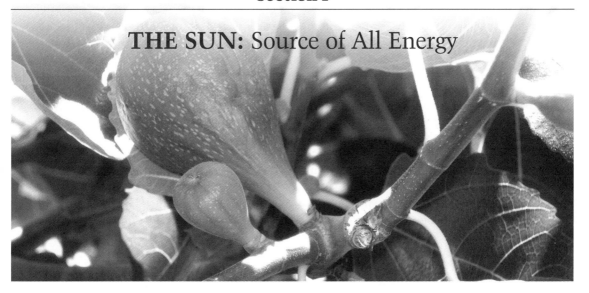

Centuries of consumer shopping have proven that you cannot shampoo health into your hair, brush health into your teeth, gargle health into your breath, smear health into your skin, pound health into your muscles, or paint health onto your face.

Health results from a balanced flow of life energy. Nutrition plays *the* key role in the production and management of that energy. Why? Because all energy on the Earth, as well as nutrition, originates from the sun. But humans and animals cannot absorb energy directly from the sun. It is the plant that converts the sun's energy into nutrients, which in turn feed our cell mitochondria to produce this dynamic life force for the body.

The plant lives by absorbing energy from the sun, then using that energy to covert inorganic substances from the soil into organic substances. It converts minerals, gases of the air (carbon dioxide and oxygen) into food. The energy is the sun's heat. Your temperature of 98 degrees is the sun's heat stored up by a plant for you to release when you eat that plant. –Dr. Royal Lee[1]

The sun's energy, stored in the plant along with phytochemicals (complex chemicals made by the plant), is liberated when the animal or human digests the plant cells. But energy from the sun cannot be transformed without chlorophyll. That's why Dr. Lee liked to say: *When you order a steak, you're eating grass.*

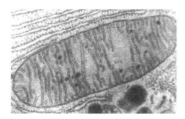

Mitochondria produce energy for the cell through cellular respiration.

Such a powerful transformation from solar energy to earth energy is rarely appreciated as the foundation for health. Today, simply saying "To improve health, eat a good diet" is not much help. The very word "diet" has come to mean whatever is being promoted as the latest fad, particularly for weight loss. We are a culture that has lost instinct and knowledge of what constitutes healthful food.

---

[1] *See Appendix, **AUDIO CD's** section,* Lectures of Dr. Royal Lee, Vol. II

What is a Good Diet?

According to the US Department of Agriculture, the average American will consume calories generated from about 50 tons of food in a lifetime. Over fifty-percent of those calories will come from refined sugars and altered, synthetic fats. After eating this way for so many years, we need (1) nutrient-rich food in place of refined food, (2) therapeutic nutritional support to restore energy and proper function to all systems in the body, and (3) an ability to recognize healthy food.

This book will help you discriminate between healthy and unhealthy sources of food. It will also tell you why the right type of nutritional supplement is necessary in today's world, and why you probably are not getting this nutrition from the food you are eating.

The health professional who recommended this book is trained and committed to help you transform your lifestyle into one that is healthy and productive, irrespective of inherent limitations. But, ultimately, each person's health is his or her personal responsibility. Using the information in this book, you can better educate yourself to make insightful choices about the foods you feed to yourself and to your loved ones.

Why Can't I Live In Wellness?

We know that machine parts wear out or break down simply from use over time, from neglect, or from abuse. However, unlike a machine, the human body can renew and regenerate itself, *if* it has what it needs. The body produces new cells every day for every organ and gland. Healing of injuries, both minor and severe, is routine. Why, then, is health so elusive?

The answer to this question lies under our feet: Health begins in the soil. It is from the soil that elements are taken up and transformed by the plant into nutrients we can assimilate. If this supply of building material and energy is not constant and balanced, our bodies wear out and break down prematurely. Unfortunately our modern mechanized world gives emphasis to quantity rather than quality of foodstuffs. Although we pride ourselves on caloric abundance, it has been demonstrated that empty calories and de-mineralized foods lead to malnutrition just as surely as no food at all.

In 1913, Major General Sir Robert McCarrison, M.D., became chief medical officer to the British troops in India. He was already a celebrated endocrine researcher, noted for his discoveries on the cause of goiter. In India, he conducted large-scale food experiments on animals. This work presented the first scientific research demonstrating that the endocrine system suffers the first lesions of malnutrition (beginning with the adrenals, then the thymus, then the thyroid), leading to degeneration throughout the body. He was recognized for this seminal work with a knighthood. In 1928, he became Director of Nutritional Research in India.

McCarrison came to his conclusions by studying a healthy people—the Hunza's—who were living in the Himalayan Mountains, in a remote region in what today is part of Pakistan. He observed and recorded how the yearly inundation of their fields—by melting glaciers—re-mineralized the soil. The alternating swelling and contraction of the glacier ground the surface of the mountain underneath it to dust. This mineral dust fed their soil every year, resulting in abundant, healthy crops and fruit trees with unusually long life spans.

McCarrison's book, *Studies in Deficiency Disease*,[2] published in 1921, documented his findings that the more minerals the soil contains, the higher the mineral, vitamin and protein content in

---

[2] *Studies in Deficiency Disease, is presently out of print and no longer in copyright. It is now in the public domain. Selene River Press offers it—at no charge—as a downloadable Acrobat file in the "Historical Archives" section of their website. See Appendix, BOOK or RESOURCES sections*

the plant. His studies influenced many others in the health professions. Dr. McCarrison's work was a foundation stone for the work of Dr. Weston A. Price whose book, *Nutrition and Physical Degeneration*, is a global survey of what happened to the health of indigenous peoples when they switched from their own diet to "the foods of commerce." McCarrison was J.I. Rodale's mentor in launching his nutritional publishing empire. And Dr. McCarrison's research greatly assisted Dr. Royal Lee's work.[3] When he was a teenager, Dr. Lee began keeping a notebook about nutrition and health, in which he recorded his theory that the endocrine system was the first system to break down from malnutrition. By 1915, Dr. Lee was convinced that this was indeed the case. McCarrison's findings, published in 1921, confirmed Lee's theory of the nutrition-endocrine connection.[4]

Devitalized and De-mineralized Foods
Result from the Following:

- farming methods that do not rejuvenate the soil

- chemical farming techniques that contaminate and sterilize the soil

- refining methods that remove or destroy nutrients from food

- the use of chemical preservatives, artificial colors and flavors that pollute food

- the use of irradiation and genetic alteration that damages the biological structure of food

- the creation of manmade junk non-foods that substitute for healthy food

- the use of agricultural and industrial toxins that contaminate food through pollution of water, air and land

---

Less than 50 years after Justice Von Liebig wrote his landmark book, Agricultural Chemistry, which forged the marriage of farming and the chemical industry in 1853, many scientists and doctors spoke out against the poisoning of the food supply. It was Rachael Carson in 1962, with her book, Silent Spring, who captured the awareness of popular culture with the visual imagery of a spring without birds. Today, agricultural pollution accounts for more pollution worldwide than all other forms of pollution added together. Rain washes the toxins into streams, rivers, oceans, and underground aquifers.

---

[3] *See Appendix, BOOKS section, for more on Price and Lee*

[4] *See "ABOUT DR. ROYAL LEE"*

The forces of heredity definitely tend to inflict upon unborn children the penalties of poor judgment and carelessness that their mothers and fathers exercised in selecting their food. These penalties accumulate, each generation paying a greater price in lost health. A race that fails to take notice of dietary problems soon dies out. Dr. Weston A. Price found in his travels and studies of primitive peoples that they had accumulated a remarkable folklore of nutritional information passed down from generation to generation. Now we can see that this is not so remarkable. The existence of the people he studies is actually dependent upon that folklore. Those families who failed to accurately transmit this information, to take the trouble to learn the necessary facts of life, dwindled into nothing. We think we are of higher intelligence, but are actually being subjected to that same test.

–Dr. Royal Lee

THE SOIL: Source of All Nutrients

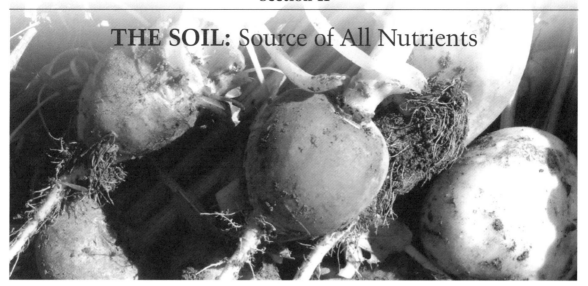

"The modern farmer treats the plant; the true farmer treats the soil."
- Mark R. Anderson

A plant is only as healthy as the soil in which it grows. Plants do not manufacture minerals; they absorb them from the soil. Plants do manufacture vitamins, proteins, fats and carbohydrates, but without minerals, the vitamins cannot function as catalysts. Mineral-deficient plants also lack both quality and quantity of proteins. *Only fertile, balanced soil yields healthy, nutritious plants, vegetables and livestock.*

What Makes Soil Fertile?

Living microbes and over thirty-two elements known as trace minerals make soil fertile. It is the organic matter in soil that provides food for the beneficial microbes. These microbes break down complex matter into more basic elements, without which the plant would starve.

Without microbes, soil ceases to be a life-giving biomass because those microbes alone facilitate the cycling of carbon, calcium, phosphorus, sulfur, and other essential minerals. Nitrogen-fixing bacteria stimulate the growth of plants, and fungi assist the transference of minerals from the soil into the plant roots. It has been estimated that one-thousand square feet of healthy topsoil contains up to 12,000 pounds of beneficial microorganisms. You can easily see why agricultural chemicals are so counterproductive in the long run: they kill soil microbes. Soil fertility is dependant upon the living bridge of microbes which connects the soil to the plant.[5]

Without trace minerals—such as copper, chromium, iron, iodine, selenium, magnesium and zinc—plants become deficient, stressed, and susceptible to disease. Most commercial farmers now use farming methods that sterilize and deplete the soil, producing weak and deficient plants. They then apply toxic chemicals to keep these sickly plants alive and force them to produce deficient fruits and vegetables. More toxic poisons are put on the Earth from agriculture than all other forms of pollution combined! It's hard work trying to ward off Nature's intelligent effort

---

[5] *See Appendix, BOOKS section,* Empty Harvest, *by Mark R. Anderson*

to destroy inferior food. Rather than entering into a partnership with Nature, the farmer has unknowingly declared war against Nature.

Trace minerals occur in such minute quantities that we measure them in parts per million. They are the basis of the complex chemical and electrical mechanism that is your body. Without them, vitamins fail to function. However, the minerals in your body and the minerals in the soil are in two different states—organic and inorganic. The inorganic minerals in soil bind with plant protein in a process called "chelation." During the growth cycle, plants transform inorganic minerals from the soil into organically-bound minerals which your body can then use.

To further illustrate this point, both kale and oyster shells are sources of calcium. Which would you rather have with your dinner? Even if you choose oyster shells, your body will know the difference and not be able to use this inorganic form of calcium. Yet many manufacturers of nutritional supplements make oyster shell calcium supplements. Knowing that, you can read labels and avoid this inorganic form of calcium.

When humans or animals digest plant protein, they absorb the minerals. However, for all these processes to occur, plants need a rich supply of trace minerals from the soil. It is no wonder we call industrial factories "plants." Nothing on Earth works as efficiently as a plant does to manufacture the sustenance of life for all other life forms. From the oxygen we breathe to the vitamins, minerals and proteins of our cells, the soil-born plant is our ultimate link to life on this planet.

Again, nutritional deficiencies begin in the soil. In order to transform the mineral kingdom into the human and animal kingdoms, the vegetable kingdom must have quality, balanced, fertile soil, rich in microbes and nutrients from organic matter. Chemically-treated, chemically-fed and chemically-contaminated foods are the harvest of starving soil. The harmful levels of chemicals such as pesticides and herbicides further diminish the bio-availability of nutrients and can lead to disease.

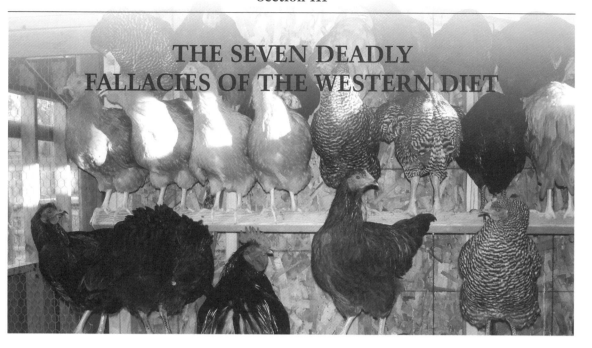

THE SEVEN DEADLY FALLACIES OF THE WESTERN DIET

The quest for superior nutrition has never been easy. Historically, it has demanded a deft combination of art and instinct, whether it is the skill of the hunter, or the wisdom of the cook. Today all we need is a driver's license to get to the grocery store! But this convenience comes with a price: the loss of fundamental skills in how to nourish ourselves and our family. **The devastating result of adopting conveniences without preserving the goal of superior nutrition can be seen in the following list:**

The Seven Deadly Fallacies of the Western Diet

- Chlorinated and fluoridated water is safe to drink.

- Grains that are processed, refined, and fortified with a few synthetic vitamins build a strong body.

- Animal and dairy fats are dangerous to your heart and vascular system, BUT synthetic fat such as hydrogenated oil, and oleo products such as margarine, are healthful.

- Refined sugar is a food.

- Pasteurized dairy is a nutritious source of minerals, vitamins and protein.

- Vegetables and fruits grown on chemically-treated soil are safe and healthy to eat.

- Animals raised in feed lots and supplemented with hormones and antibiotics are a safe, healthy food source.

Here are some of the facts that expose these fallacies, facts you need in order to make informed choices about your diet and health.

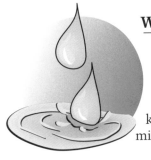

WATER

Water does much more than quench our thirst. In fact, it is one of the most important factors in maintaining equilibrium of the various body systems. Of course it is hydrating, but it is also essential for lubricating, cleansing, transporting nutrients and regulating temperature. Would it surprise you to know water is a source of nutrients, providing important minerals and trace minerals?

Water comprises 70 percent of the adult body weight. The human brain is composed of 95 percent water; blood is 82 percent water; the lungs are nearly 90 percent water. You can live for about a month without food, but only about a week without water. The human body is constantly losing water through sweat, urine, and breathing.

When we drink water—as with all food—quality matters. Because the goal of every living creature is to select food and water that will prevent deficiency diseases and poisoning, it stands to reason that, *"Any poison added to food or drink is too much. Like emery powder in a gear box, the damage is proportional to the amount and shortens life accordingly."* –Dr. Royal Lee

Some of the daily concerns about drinking water are the additives—chlorine, fluoride and water softeners—and toxic agricultural runoff such as nitrates and nitrites. If you do not have a source of clean well or spring water running through your tap, then research the right water purification system to remove pollutants from your water. Water purification systems should be tailored to the kind of water problems in your location. Local water districts, at your request, will give you an analysis of your water.[6]

Chlorine—an oxidizing chemical bleach—is one of the most toxic substances on earth. Along with killing dangerous bacteria in water, it can destroy healthy intestinal flora, primarily healthy bacteria. This destruction allows resistant pathogenic bacteria an opportunity to flourish within our gastro-intestinal (GI) tract. Healthy bacterial flora is part of the body's first line of defense against ingested pathogens. The healthful and friendly bacteria in the intestines not only further break down our food for absorption, they deprive harmful bacteria and fungi the opportunity to take up residence and poison the body. Without healthy intestinal flora to aid in proper digestion, the body is starved of nutrients needed for growth, repair and defense. The symptoms of this deprivation make up a long and painful list.

If you are not yet suspicious of chemical additives in drinking water, consider this: If you buy fish for a fresh water aquarium, you will have to de-chlorinate the water or the first thing your fish will do is...die! You also have to replace some of the bacteria which the chlorine has destroyed. Naturally occurring bacteria in water, known as "pyrogens," have an antigenic effect for all living creatures. (Antigens stimulate an immune response.)

Although the immune-building quality of water deserves a great deal more research, pyrogenic bacteria is another fascinating property of natural spring water which Dr. Lee wrote about in a 1958 article for *Let's Live Magazine*:

Good water is water that has been filtered through the ground to reach the well or spring and has thereby accumulated a load of antigens. These antigens are otherwise known to

---

[6] *See Appendix, WATER section*

science as "pyrogens," since they cause fever if injected into the bloodstream. They are the residue of disease-producing bacteria, and by drinking them we develop an immunity to the germ or virus that put them into the water. In foreign countries where polio is relatively nonexistent as a known disease, the bloodstream of the children has been found loaded with antibodies to polio, which prevented them from contracting the disease. These children were immunized the natural way, not by a shot of Salk vaccine. It is very probable that their diet of unrefined natural foods that promptly supplies the necessary factors to make antibodies was responsible for their freedom from polio.[7]

Just when we slip into dismissing earlier research as being unsupported by modern research, science re-discovers some piece of the earlier research. For instance, following is an excerpt from the Scripts Howard News Service reporting on a study in the professional science journal *Cell*, dated April 2004, titled, "Driven to Autoimmunity: the NOD Mouse:"

"Scientists at The Scripps Research Institute in La Jolla, Calif., said they were able to boost the supply of critical T cells and curtail development of insulin-dependent diabetes in mice genetically cued to develop the autoimmune disease. The team, led by immunologist Nora Sarvetnick, reported a surge in the T-cell count when the mice were challenged with a mixture of bacterial cell-wall components. 'Autoimmunity has been considered a condition of too much stimulation,' Sarvetnick said. 'What we are seeing is that it is a condition of too little stimulation.'

"Sarvetnick and her team said their theory would explain why childhood bacterial infections decrease the risk for developing autoimmune diseases like Type 1 diabetes, rheumatoid arthritis, lupus and even asthma, and why incidence of these diseases has been on the rise in less-germ-tolerant, developed countries during the past 50 years compared to less-developed nations. 'The cleaner everyone is, the less stimulation their immune system gets,' Sarvetnick said. 'Their immune system tends to be incomplete."

Another common additive to drinking water is fluoride.[8] Fluoride is medically categorized as protoplasmic poison, which is why it is used to kill rodents. There are many studies proving the toxicity of fluoride as well as its unfounded use in dental health. This subject is well worth looking into further, as are the effects of drinking water contaminated with pesticides and herbicides.[9]

Water softeners work by de-mineralizing—particularly de-calcifying—the water through the use of salt. Minerals, such as calcium bicarbonate, are what make water hard and are one of the reasons, in addition to hydration, we need to drink water. Calcium bicarbonate is a form of calcium that is completely assimilated. It builds bone by combining with the organic phosphorus found in food and the lecithins of natural fats. The use of water softeners is another act of turning healthy water into a refined food. Also, the salt used in this process is flushed into the ground water, harming the environment. The salt gives water a slippery, slimy feel, making additional filtration necessary before consuming.

The unique forms of minerals in water—such as calcium bicarbonate—and immune-stimulating bacteria in water cause us to realize **water is another form of food for the body**, not just a void, thirst-quenching liquid. The only good thing about distilled water, for instance, is that it's wet. Therefore, it is vital that we obtain water that is intact rather than refined and stripped of its nutrients.

---

[7] *See Appendix, ARTICLES section, "Ideal Drinking Water," by Dr. Royal Lee, Let's Live Magazine*

[8] *See Appendix, FLUORIDE section*

[9] *See Appendix, WATER HEALTH section*

GRAINS

Astonishing as it may be, grains that have been grown on depleted soil, fed chemical fertilizer, and sprayed with toxic herbicides and pesticides are ***then*** stripped of most of their nutrients for shipping and preserving purposes! Such processing includes the commercial refinement of whole wheat berries which removes the bran (fiber and nutrients) and germ (the most nutritionally-dense portion), leaving the starch we call "flour." The precious bran and germ are fed to animals, because they are known to produce strong, healthy stock! Refining the grain would be a great idea ***if*** the most significant nutritional value of wheat were not in the bran and germ. But both wheat bran and germ contain fiber, vitamins B and E, and minerals. There are some minerals left in the starch. But, without the bran and the germ in the starch, the body cannot absorb them properly.

Freshly milled grains contain fats and oils that are as perishable as any other raw food. People accustomed to buying packaged flour do not realize that freshly ground flour is one of the most perishable foods in the world, no different from an apple which, when sliced open, soon turns brown. Oxidation is what turns oils in flour rancid. An experienced miller can taste flour and tell how many hours ago it was ground. To overcome this obstacle in the commercial market, chlorine-derived chemical bleaches are used to strip the remaining oils. This process preserves the flour, but leaves toxic chemical residues in every bite. Then several synthetically-made chemical vitamins are sprayed into the flour.

If food were a dead substance, it wouldn't spoil. Instead of finding ways to keep people fed properly, the very beauty of living food is perceived as an inconvenience. Nevertheless, the inescapable fact remains that a living body needs living food, the only source of the living nourishment that builds living cells and living tissue. How, then, can we justify the processing of living food into substances that rob us of our health?

Fortunately, the marketplace has responded to the need for nutritious food. Whole grains, organically grown on chemical-free soil, are available in most health food stores. These include grains such as wheat, brown rice, millet, rye, oats, buckwheat, yellow and blue corn, spelt, amaranth and quinoa. With a good quality, home flour mill you can mill grains right before baking or cooking, which is the only way to avoid oxidation and guaranty freshness.[10]

Because it is highly perishable, flour should be used within twenty minutes of being ground. However, there is another element to consider when eating grains. Author Sally Fallon teaches in her book, *Nourishing Traditions*, that our ancestors in their non-industrialized societies had the wisdom to know that grains have to be prepared properly in order for us to digest them.[11]

Here is an excerpt from Sally Fallon's *Nourishing Traditions*:

> *We recommend the use of a variety of whole grains but with an important caveat. Phosphorus in the bran of whole grains is tied up in a substance called phytic acid. Phytic acid combines with iron, calcium, magnesium, copper and zinc in the intestinal tract, blocking their absorption. Whole grains also contain enzyme inhibitors that can interfere with digestion. Traditional societies usually soak or ferment their grains before eating them, processes that neutralize phytates and enzyme inhibitors and, in effect, predigest grains so that all their nutrients are more available. Sprouting, overnight soaking and old-fashioned sour leavening can accomplish this important pre-digestion in our own kitchens. Many people*

---

[10] *See Appendix, FLOUR MILLS section*

[11] *See Appendix, BOOKS section*

who are allergic to grains will tolerate them well when they are prepared according to these procedures. Proper preparation techniques also help break down complex sugars in legumes, making them more digestible. –Sally Fallon, *Nourishing Traditions*

Properly grown and prepared, whole grains will add high quality vitamins, minerals, proteins and fiber to your diet. It is no surprise that many people are now allergic to grains when we have abandoned the age-old wisdom of how to prepare them for proper digestion.

FATS and OILS

Next time you're in the shower, ask yourself why your skin is water repellant. Healthy skin is rich in natural oils. Oil (essential fats) will repel water. Healthy skin is also able to retain moisture from the inside. You will notice if your skin is not retaining moisture well, or if you're bothered by skin and scalp conditions. These conditions may be caused by a deficiency of the essential fatty acids. Many food authorities have proven that consumption of hydrogenated oils and oleo products, such as margarine and processed commercial cooking oils, aggravates this problem. In fact, the government now requires food processing companies to list the hydrogenated oil content on their labels rather than disguising it within the listing of total fats.

Why do manufacturers hydrogenate oil? Essential fatty acids go rancid in the presence of air. So manufacturers look for cheap ways to process, ship and preserve the shelf-life of oil. By exposing the oil to hydrogen gas and a catalyst (nickel) at high temperatures and pressures, the oil molecule is broken down and reassembled into new forms, in this case saturated with hydrogen, which raises the melting point. After refining, bleaching and deodorizing, this synthetic fat is re-flavored and re-colored.

However, we cannot benefit nutritionally from hydrogenated fats because the liver has difficulty converting them into forms the body is designed to use. To the degree the fat you eat is hydrogenated, you are contributing to vitamin deficiency, elevated blood cholesterol, and liver toxicity. These effects can set the stage for blood, heart, gland, and skin disorders. That is why using fresh, unrefined oils and fats which provide a rich supply of essential fatty acids is so important. Meanwhile, hydrogenation makes the grocer happy because the hydrogenated fat lasts a long time on the shelf, and the manufacturer is happy because he does not have to be concerned about spoilage in shipping. Good for the manufacturer, good for the grocer, **bad** for your present and future health.

To avoid these toxic oils, and because of erroneous weight concerns, many people have mistakenly sought to eliminate all oils and fats from their diet. This mistake could lead to tragic consequences. Vitamins A, E, D, K and essential fatty acids—necessary for glandular and organ health—are lost in such an approach. For example, fat soluble vitamin E is essential to the production of hormones during puberty. Loss of this vitamin leads to endocrine, skin and heart trouble.

Unrefined oils such as sesame, olive ("extra virgin" indicates the olive oil is unrefined), grape seed, peanut oil, tropical oils such as coconut oil and red palm oil, and foods such as fish, healthy meat, fresh sweet cream butter and sesame tahini, are excellent sources of the essential fatty acids.[12] NOTE: "Cold-processed" alone does not necessarily mean the oil is unrefined or has been processed at low temperatures.[13]

---

[12] *See* Nourishing Traditions *by Sally Fallon for a clear, concise lesson in fats and oils*

[13] *See Appendix, BOOKS section,* Food Fundamentals, *by Judith DeCava*

It is important to read labels, *especially* in health food stores because we tend to let our guard down, assuming if it's being sold in a health food store, it must be healthful. Unfortunately, that is not the case.[14] Be on the lookout for hydrogenated oils, as well as foods containing hydrogenated oil, including those that are "partially hydrogenated." Margarine, commercial cooking oils, and other processed foods such as commercial peanut butter, in most instances, are made from hydrogenated oils.

It is well-worth the effort to learn about the varieties of oils and fats available, and the difference between safe and unsafe processing methods.[15] For example, in the "US EPA Biopesticide Decision Document: Canola Oil," issued October 1998, canola oil is registered as an EPA approved biochemical insecticide. Yet, the EPA deems it safe for consumption. It is made from rape seed oil that has been genetically-engineered and irradiated. The rape plant is the most toxic of all food oil plants—not even insects will eat it. It is a member of the mustard family, and is the source for the chemical agent, mustard gas. First developed in Canada, and re-named Canadian Oil, canola oil is industrial oil. Some of its uses are as a lubricant, fuel, soap, and synthetic rubber base.

> "During the deodorizing process, the omega-3 fatty acids of processed canola oil are transformed into *trans* fatty acids, similar to those in margarine and possibly more dangerous. A recent study indicates that "heart healthy" canola oil actually creates a deficiency of vitamin E, a vitamin required for a healthy cardiovascular system. Other studies indicate that even low-erucic-acid canola oil causes heart lesions, particularly when the diet is also low in saturated fat." –Sally Fallon, *Nourishing Traditions*

Erroneous weight concerns have played a serious role in turning us away from the highly concentrated source of nutrition in fats. Fats remain an irreplaceable source of nutrients and energy. Fat-soluble vitamins such as A, D, E, F, and K feed the eyes, liver, heart, skin and bones. Foods that concentrate these vitamins most efficiently come from animal sources: eggs, butter, fish liver oil, animal organs (especially liver), and raw (unpasteurized) dairy products. The survival of all mammals depends upon the ability of the mother to concentrate these nutrients within her own cells and pass them along— through her raw milk—to her offspring. Animal food, in the form of milk, is the first food given to every mammal because it provides the greatest chances for survival as well as for its future health.

Fat provides a much slower and more efficient burning of energy in contrast to the quick depletion resulting from refined sugars and refined carbohydrates. Animals that hibernate, for example, are efficiently liberating energy from fat. A diet high in refined carbohydrates, such as refined flours and sugars, combined with a low energy demand, results in an excess of glucose which the body must store. In order to store it, the body creates fat cells and triglycerides. But unaltered fat consumed from healthy animals or oils triggers the fat combustion ("burning") process in the body.

SWEETS AND SWEETENERS

Natural, unrefined sugars do not cause extremes of imbalance the way refined sugars do. They provide an energy that burns slower and more evenly. Interestingly, the carbohydrate form of energy is not essential to a state of health because the body can extract glucose for energy from healthy fats and proteins. This is a fact proven by Dr. Weston Price and his studies of indigenous people who lived in perfect health on only animal and fish sources of fats and proteins.[16] A reasonably healthy person can also maintain balance with unrefined complex carbohydrates such as grains, vegetables, and fruits.

---

[14] *See Section VIII "Beware of False Profits: Navigating in a Health Food Store"*

[15] *See* Know Your Fats: The Complete Primer for Understanding the Nutrition of Fats, Oils and Cholesterol *by Mary G. Enig*

[16] *See Appendix, BOOKS section,* Nutrition and Physical Degeneration, *by Dr. Weston A. Price*

However, having something sweet has always been a treat for all ages in our need for comfort and sensuousness. Many minerals such as iron, potassium and phosphorous are present in natural unrefined sweeteners such as raw, unrefined sugarcane (found as Muscavado or Rapadura), grade B or C maple syrup, raw honey, unsulfured blackstrap molasses, carob powder, fresh fruit, unsulfured dried fruit, and whole herb Stevia.

Now for the bad news: Refined cane and beet sugar, filtered maple syrup, and pasteurized honey do not contain the nutrients they did in their unrefined state. For example, sugarcane processing removes all the nutrients except for the sucrose, a simple carbohydrate constituting less than 1 percent of the whole sugarcane plant. Although it is well known that refined sugar consumption contributes to tooth decay, there is a particularly interesting study that was made in the Philippines. The city of Manila had a very high use of refined, white sugar. There was also a corresponding high incidence of tooth decay. On the sugar plantations outside the city, where the workers chewed raw sugarcane stalks throughout the day, tooth decay was rare. Why? The minerals and protective factors in raw cane juice are useful to the body and aid it to properly process the sugars. Conversely, sucrose—separated from the rest of the elements in sugarcane—stresses the body's ability to effectively handle and metabolize sugar. Countless studies and doctors' reports reveal white table sugar is an anti-nutrient that can adversely alter energy metabolism and cause nutritional deficiencies.[17]

When reading labels, know the synonyms used to describe refined sugar: cane sugar, beet sugar, sucrose, glucose, corn syrup, turbinado sugar and brown sugar (white sugar with molasses added).[18]

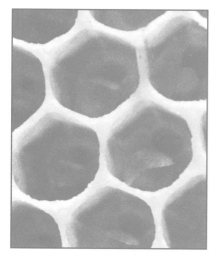

Truly raw honey[19] is extracted by centrifugal force. Heat can be used so long as it is under 100° F, otherwise some of the living constituents and enzymes will be destroyed. Pasteurization is considered complete at 143° F. In warm climates, honey will be liquid and will not crystallize. But all honey will crystallize in cooler temperatures, even in the hive. It will crystallize more readily if it contains components of the hive. But if not, it will crystallize if kept cool (about 57°). If both blended and stored at cool temperatures, it will crystallize more quickly.

Honey can be strained and liquid in a raw state. But if it has been fine- or ultra-filtered, it has been heated and is not considered raw. It can also be liquid and not strained, again, if it is in a warm climate.

"When talking about honey, it's advisable to buy unpasteurized honey, because pasteurized honey is just as bad as pasteurized milk. It's a natural food, and even after it's pasteurized it won't decalcify your bones like sugar will, but it won't give you the vitamins. If you feed pasteurized honey to bees it will kill them.

I have a letter from the Department of Agriculture to whom we wrote in and asked if it was safe to feed bees on cooked honey, the kind you buy in the store. It's all cooked, you know, to keep it from crystallizing in the jar. They said "No, don't ever think of it because it will kill the bees." So, that's the situation. We're eating food that's destroyed. Its food value is gone by simple-minded processing, processing that is totally unnecessary if we realized the

---

[17]See Appendix, BOOKS section, Sugar Blues, by William Dufty

[18] See Appendix, BOOKS section, Food Fundamentals, by Judith DeCava, for a more comprehensive list

[19] See Appendix, FOOD SOURCES section

consequences. It's just a convenience to the processor. He puts his honey on the grocery store shelf, and the customer objects to buying it if it's crystallized.

Now let me give you a tip about crystallized honey. The only thing that crystallizes in honey is the glucose, natural glucose. If you take a jar of crystallized honey and turn it upside down over a plate with a couple of supports across, to let the honey drain out and let it stand maybe a week (it takes a week before it quits dripping out), you will find that the glucose crystals that are left are absolutely repulsive to the sense of taste. You wouldn't think of eating it. Bees won't eat it. And if you dissolve that in water and feed it to your bees they will die. The valuable part of that honey is all in the fluid part that did not crystallize and which can be drained off and used. And you'll find that it is twice as sweet as the original honey. And another thing, the diabetic can use that drained off sweet and will find that he'll get no adverse affect on his blood sugar. So there are some interesting things about honey. Even honey, natural honey, has too much glucose and we'd be better off getting rid of it. And the bees are better off getting rid of it.

If you want to accelerate this crystallization you could stir up the honey a bit and then put it away. In fact, if you put it in a food mixer and start stirring it, it will crystallize inside of twenty minutes. You'll get a honey butter. Well if you put that butter away in a jar, the crystals will grow bigger and then in a few weeks you can tip it upside down and drain off your honey. If the honey doesn't come out when you invert it, it's because you're trying to drain it off before the crystals have gotten big enough to allow the non-crystallized part to separate. But the part that does not crystallize is the valuable and healthful part. And the crystals themselves, after you've drained off the liquid, are nothing but pure glucose and are not suitable for food."

–Dr. Royal Lee, *Lectures of Dr. Royal Lee Volume II*

MILK

If you drink milk, the most nutritious milk is certified Grade-A raw. It can be a healthful addition to the diet because it provides one of the few sources of raw and total protein. In addition, dairy products made from raw milk are excellent sources of nutrition for all ages. The aging and fermentation processes applied in the making of cheese, kefir, or yogurt, for instance, make the milk completely digestible. Fermented foods are also an important source of intestinal flora, adding to the body's strength of digestion and cleansing.

Advertising makes much of drinking milk for its calcium. But the raw milk enzyme, *phosphatase*, is destroyed by the temperatures of pasteurization—and phosphatase is the very enzyme required for calcium to bond to bone! Pasteurization kills *all* the living enzyme systems, making pasteurized milk difficult to digest. Many doctors have noted that allergies and constipation may result.[20] Dr. Royal Lee and Dr. Francis Pottenger taught that arthritis and degenerative bone syndromes were "cooked foods diseases" in which the heat-labile essential amino acids are removed from the diet through over-cooking. Without the essential amino acids, the collagen connective tissue degenerates, and the body's immune system breaks it down.

If Nature provides such a valuable food, why do we destroy its value through pasteurization? Pasteurization allows farmers to sell unsanitary milk to dairies, where it will be heat-sterilized.

---

[20] *See Section IV, PROFESSIONAL GUIDANCE: The Digestive System*

Sterilizing it disguises the lack of cleanliness.

Raw milk would provide us with an abundant source of intact amino acids, unaltered fats, minerals and vitamins. Unfortunately raw milk is illegal in some states, not on nutritional grounds, but for fear of contamination. This fear has been proven unfounded, a conclusion which is documented on the Weston A. Price Foundation website. It is well worth your effort to look for sources of raw milk in your area.[21]

Milk is also homogenized. Homogenization breaks down the fat molecules so the cream content is no longer visible. A high cream content indicates high quality milk. Homogenization allows the producer to mix all grades of milk together, removing any incentive for the farmer to produce high quality milk. Also, homogenization can lead to illegal practices such as combining outdated milk with fresh milk for resale.

For adults who have no allergies or sensitivities to dairy products, moderate amounts of milk by-products are much better: butter, yogurt and aged hard cheese. Seed and nut milks are tasty, nutritious alternatives to milk, and were used by many robust indigenous people for centuries when animal milk was not available.

VEGETABLES and FRUITS

Back to Nature's factory: the plant. In all the food categories, is there a wider variety of goodness and healing than you find in the plant kingdom? From flowers to herbs, the plant kingdom is highly innovative: flowers can be prepared homeopathically, blended in perfumes, eaten raw in salad and brewed as tea; herbs can be prepared medicinally, used in culinary arts, and brewed as beer!

We have already discussed the need to start with healthy soil from which the plant can take up an abundance of nutrients and transform them from the inorganic to the organic state. In fact, it is the nutrient content of a vegetable or fruit that gives it flavor. Just because it looks like a carrot doesn't mean it tastes like one or delivers the nourishment a carrot should. When vegetables are grown on depleted soil, if they have any flavor at all, they might taste sweet, but they don't usually have the full, concentrated, complexity of flavors derived from microbial, nutrient rich soil. Is it any wonder why kids don't want to eat their vegetables?

Just as human malnutrition invites disease, so does malnutrition in the soil cause insect, fungal, and bacterial disease in plants. The first sign of a healthy plant is it can survive without the aid of drugs.

In his book, *Empty Harvest*, Mark R. Anderson[22] describes in detail the connection between the soil and the human immune system. He documents how people, who once farmed according to this connection, kept their civilizations free of diseases that are now common in today's world. Fortunately, organic farming and gardening methods are easily accessible to us. All the shopping in the best food markets cannot substitute for your own experience of growing vegetables and fruits. Make yourself a small plot of dirt and plant some seeds. Even potted lettuce, tomatoes and herbs will grow well in any sunny location and can be moved around easily. Beautiful, whole food, fresh and vibrant from the air, sun and soil, is what it's all about.

---

[21] *See Appendix, BOOKS and FOOD SOURCES sections*

[22] *See Appendix, BOOKS section*

MEAT

Vegetarians often claim that animal products shorten life span, while some meat eaters wonder if a vegetarian diet can possibly be healthy. Arguments in favor of either can be made and supported. For example, here is an observation about the benefits of meat:

Russians from the Caucasus Mountains, an area famous for longevity, eat fatty meat and whole milk products frequently. Studies of Soviet Georgian populations show that those who have the most meat and fat in their diets live the longest. Inhabitants of Vilcabamba in Ecuador, known for their longevity, consume a variety of animal foods including whole milk and fatty pork. The long-lived people of Hunza consume animal protein in the form of high-fat goat milk products. On the other hand, the vegetarian inhabitants of southern India have one of the shortest life spans in the world.
–Sally Fallon, *Nourishing Traditions*

The research represented in the previous quote is but a fraction from a large body of research demonstrating that animal meat and fat in the diet provides the highest quality and greatest concentration of nutrients necessary for health. However, indigenous people ate meat that was (1) only lightly cooked (preserving the integrity of proteins), and (2) raised in the wild, or free-range, on soil, water and land that was unpolluted by toxic chemicals. And they ate the glands, organs, and cartilage (gristle), which contain an even higher concentration of nutrients than the flesh. The amount and quality of nutrients in such meat is hard to beat. But some people—perhaps because of the difficulty and expense of obtaining healthy meat, or because of poor digestion, or for philosophical reasons—look to a vegetarian diet and have been successful in creating one that works for them. We each have to discover and respect our biochemical individuality.[23]

Also, indigenous people did not eat protein in highly denatured states such as occurs with overcooking, over-processing, and hydrolyzing. Hydrolyzed soy protein, for example, is often an ingredient in protein powders. Rather than using this substance as a high-quality protein, the body actually uses most of it as a sugar.

The central point is this: If you consume meat, it must be healthy meat. Know the source of the meat and how it was raised. When you invest in a computer or a car, for instance, you make it your business to know the manufacturer's reputation. So it must be with meat. Increasingly, organic meat producers are putting their names on their products and maintaining websites to inform customers of their philosophies and methods of animal husbandry. [24]

Meat is another food that is worth raising yourself, even if it's just a few chickens or a goat. When you "get up close and personal" with the life that will nurture you and your family, eating is restored to the sacred act it was meant to be. For one thing, it would be much more difficult to knowingly apply toxic substances to the food you feed to your children. But people often cringe at the thought of eating an animal they've come to know. It makes us feel sad to kill a creature we've raised. And it should. It should make us feel many things, such as humble in the face of such ultimate sacrifice. If we close our eyes to these facts of life, we are protecting ourselves from feeling any connection to the animal. But to raise a creature for food is to experience deep respect and humility for the gift of life in all forms.

Granted, raising animals for meat might not be an option for you. Instead, you might want to consider raising chickens for eggs, or a cow for milk, bees for honey, or a fruit tree. In any case,

---

[23] *See Appendix, ARTICLES section, "Food Fights, Part I and II," by Judith DeCava*

[24] *See Appendix, RESOURCES section*

raising your own food and knowing what you're putting into your family's bodies makes it easier to appreciate the need to keep the food free of toxins and rich in nutrients. But if raising food is not an option, a great way to get more personal with plants and animals is to get involved in Community Supported Agriculture.[25] Or perhaps a local farmer or rancher would be happy to have some volunteer help now and then. One of the quickest ways to check for a CSA farm where you live is to go to **www.google.com** and type in the following search query exactly as follows: "community supported agriculture" + *your state*.

Example:
"community supported agriculture" + Ohio yielded 6,800 hits on Google.

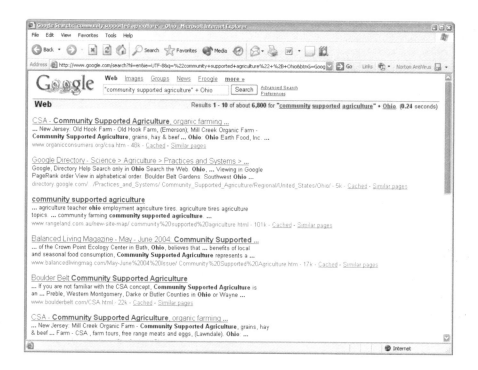

Now that we have considered each of the Seven Deadly Fallacies of the Western Diet, we hope you can see why high-quality nutritional supplements are necessary: We are starving our bodies of the very substances that food is designed to carry to every cell. While nutritional supplements—made from healthy food grown on healthy soil—play an important role in restoring us to balance, it is our hope that you are inspired to investigate further what you can do to restore delicious, healthy food to your table.

---

[25] *See Appendix, RESOURCES section*

"We tend to have sodium deficiency when we do not include enough table salt in our diet. This is aggravated in hot weather when perspiration losses further deplete sodium reserves. Herbivorous animals need extra salt to compensate for the high potassium intake in vegetables, "salt licks" being evidence of their need. Children deprived of salt have been known to crave soup (sodium oleate) because of its sodium content.

Sodium compounds in any other form than sodium chloride—ordinary table salt—may be detrimental. This same sodium chloride (table salt) is now available in a natural form of sea salt at all health food stores, and is preferred to the pure product because it contains many naturally associated trace elements. However, one should obtain a low-heat processed sea salt, as heat-treated sea salt will not support life. For example, salt water fish cannot live in water to which heat-treated sea salt has been added, but can live in water with low-heat-processed sea salt. This is just one of the many unsuspected detrimental effects when heat processes are used.

Sodium chloride is an essential constituent of the body fluids. We cannot eliminate water by osmotic transfers—we cannot perspire, our kidneys cannot eliminate waste materials and poisons—without the help of salt. Therefore, it is important that we use it in the best form. However, it must not be allowed to take the place of potassium which is the more important mineral from a physiological viewpoint

Include in your daily diet plenty of raw vegetables and, if possible, at least a glass of raw vegetable juice per day. Organic, low-heat processed sea salt should be the salt seasoning for your foods, used in amounts which are compatible with the taste and, for individuals ordinarily considered healthy, need not be restricted as to amount. Do not forget that the body cannot make something out of nothing and the human body needs sodium and potassium for its normal functioning."

– **Dr. Royal Lee, Let's Live Magazine, 1958**

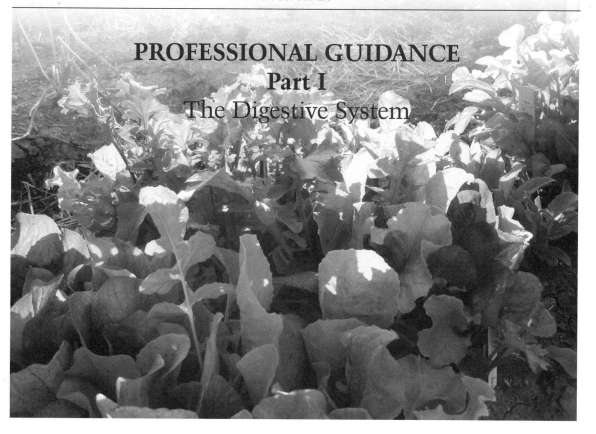

PROFESSIONAL GUIDANCE
Part I
The Digestive System

Eating healthy food is the first step toward health. The next step is seeing to it that the body has optimal ability to digest and metabolize that food. Fortunately, healthy food is much easier to digest and assimilate, especially when properly prepared so that the enzyme systems are intact. Your doctor or health professional will identify supplements you might need to assist digestion, assimilation and absorption of food.

Many times we hear that people believe they are on a balanced diet. They are even taking multiple supplements, but are still not feeling well. It may be frustrating to learn that, to the degree your digestion is inefficient and impaired, a fine diet and high quality natural supplements will not accomplish their purpose. Your doctor can suggest the right digestive supplements to correct poor digestion.

What is Digestion?

Digestion is a process during which gastric juices and enzymes break down foods into their essential and basic components: *vitamins, minerals, enzymes, amino acids, essential fatty acids, trace elements, and other organic complexes.*

A healthy digestive tract is the first line of immune defense to keep pathogens from entering the body. For instance, the stomach washes all ingested matter in a hydrochloric acid bath, which not only breaks down our food for good nutrition, but kills dangerous microbes like bacteria, fungus, and parasites. Intestinal flora, as mentioned earlier, further breaks down food for absorption.

Efficient digestion depends on the following:

- Good mastication (chewing your food), requiring healthy gums and teeth

- High enzyme content in food

- Proper hydrochloric acid and pepsin levels in the stomach

- Quality digestive enzyme production by the pancreas

- Healthy liver and gall bladder function

- Balance of proper intestinal flora (type of healthy bacterial colonies)

- Toned peristaltic action (the rhythmic motion) in the intestinal tract

- Autonomic nervous system balance

Correcting Indigestion

You cannot watch a TV program or open a magazine without seeing advertising for the drug most widely used in North America—the antacid. These products are **NOT** digestive aids as advertised because they do not aid digestion. Instead they are indigestive relief! They merely provide relief from the unpleasant symptoms of indigestion by neutralizing the acids that result from indigestion (food rotting and putrefying in the stomach). Unfortunately, they also neutralize what little digestive acid the stomach is still able to produce. In this way, antacids can impair absorption of vital nutrients such as vitamin B12 and iron. Their popularity proves that, broadly speaking, we are not digesting our food and, therefore, purchase drugs to relieve the effects of indigestion: gas, bloating, belching and heartburn. Following these symptoms, it is well known that the next problem will be constipation or diarrhea, which chronically afflicts most North Americans.

For example, iron, the anti-anemia mineral, is not absorbable in an alkaline medium. Therefore, without proper hydrochloric acid secretion in the stomach, iron absorption into the blood is greatly impaired. Antacids neutralize hydrochloric acid, and they produce an alkaline medium in the stomach. If a person is taking antacids every day for relief from poor digestion, various forms of anemia may develop. Also, when food leaves the stomach it should be in a semi-liquid state. If it is still in a mostly solid state when it enters the small intestine, the pancreatic enzymes cannot break it down enough for complete digestion and assimilation. Proteins that are not properly broken down ferment and putrefy in the intestinal tract, causing gas, bloating, toxicity and, quite often, allergies.

A great deal of digestive grief can be addressed by preparing food properly, such as soaking grains, fermenting vegetables, and souring milk. But for those whose digestion has been impaired, there are some therapeutic methods to consider. Your health professional can offer the right type of digestive aid supplements to ensure that you get the most out of what you eat. These could include digestive enzymes, acidophilus, hydrochloric acid tablets, special blends of herbs and enzymes.

Part II
The Immune System

Although we constantly hear about the "immune system," no such entity exists as a single system in the way that we have a digestive system, endocrine system, or a respiratory system. Rather, what is meant when we speak of the immune system is the natural defense reaction created by what we might call an ***alliance*** of systems. In essence, this alliance is designed to recognize anything that does not belong in the body, track it down, and eliminate it.

The immune system expresses an intelligence, creativity and self-preservation of unparalleled proportion. This multi-dimensional defense system includes the liver, thymus, spleen, the blood, the skeletal system, the digestive system, lymphatic organs, the nervous system, and parts of the endocrine system. Like a city, there is no single "Protection Department." Rather, the alliance of police, firefighters, rescue teams, ambulances, and hospitals all react and respond according to various situations, just as different immune reactions routinely occur in our body.

Although there are additional activities that the immune system performs, general references to the immune system refer, for the most part, to its ability to identify, engulf and get rid of toxins, poisons, abnormal or foreign substances, dead tissues, and wastes.

The Allies

- **Tonsils:** Collections of lymph tissue in the back of the throat; trap elements that participate in infection or inflammation.

- **Liver:** White blood cells, called leukocytes, remove harmful toxins and abnormal particulates from the blood as it filters through the liver.

- **Thymus gland:** An endocrine gland which produces new white blood cells called T-Lymphocytes (the T is for thymus) which attack foreign substances (antigens) in the blood or tissues.

- **Spleen:** Filters out abnormal cells from the blood.

- **Lymph nodes:** Filters abnormal organisms from lymph fluid and produces antibodies to eliminate bacteria, viruses, or other undesirable particulates.

- **Bone marrow:** The creation of all immune-related cells begins in the bone marrow, from where they are then released into circulation for further development by organs like the Thymus gland.

- **Mucous membranes:** The body's inner skin, which covers the respiratory, digestive, genital, and urinary tracts, prevents organisms like allergens from entering through their barrier. They contain immunoglobulins (a type of antibody) to break down such organisms.

- **Skin:** Provides a barrier that prevents organisms and allergens from entering the body.

- **Intestinal flora and stomach hydrochloric acid:** The GI Tract uses friendly bacteria and yeast to digest food and deprive harmful organisms from establishing a living colony in the digestive tract. In addition to breaking down our food, hydrochloric acid in the stomach kills many ingested parasites and bacteria.

The Immune System Alliance

TONSILS	LIVER	THYMUS	SPLEEN	LYMPHATICS
VITAMIN C, VITAMIN A, CALCIUM	B VITAMINS, VITAMINS C and K, ESSENTIAL FATTY ACIDS, WHEAT GERM OIL and WHEAT GERM	VITAMIN C, VITAMIN A, COPPER, ZINC	CHLOROPHYLL (FAT SOLUBLE), IRON, VITAMIN B12, FOLIC ACID, VITAMIN K	FLAX SEED OIL, OMEGA 3 FATTY ACIDS, FISH OILS, COD LIVER OIL, VITAMIN C

BONE MARROW	SKIN	GI FLORA	MUCOUS MEMBRANES
FOLIC ACID, VITAMIN C, AMINO ACIDS	VITAMINS A and E, SEA SALT, AMINO ACIDS, ESSENTIAL FATTY ACIDS, ZINC	ACIDOPHILUS BACTERIA, BIFIDUS BACTERIA, SOUR MILK, YOGURT, FERMENTED FOODS	VITAMIN A, C, and E, CALCIUM, ESSENTIAL FATTY ACIDS

Clearly, strengthening the immune system is fundamental to strengthening the whole body. Your doctor or health professional will employ analytical methods to determine what whole food nutrition and supplements you need to build and strengthen immunity.

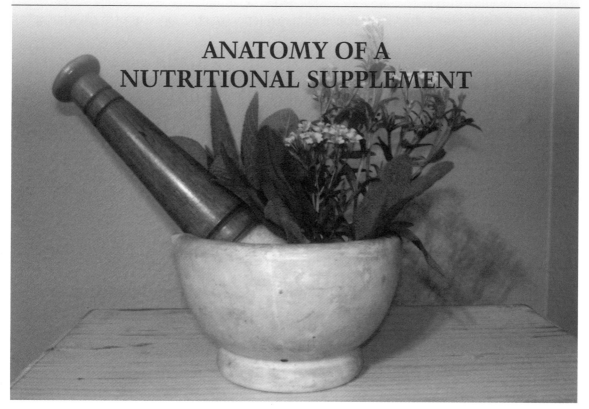

ANATOMY OF A NUTRITIONAL SUPPLEMENT

If the planting, protecting and shipping of whole foods requires extreme care and effort, imagine how much more is required to protect and preserve the nutritional quality of a concentrated food supplement. If the manufacturer's commitment to quality is not foremost, then there is no reason to swallow their pill. From the ground up, how a nutritional supplement is built will determine if it will have the desired therapeutic nutritional effect, or if it will cause more problems in the long term.

Evaluating a Nutritional Supplement

- Does the label list the foods that are concentrated?

- Are the foods organically grown and in the peak of freshness when processed?

- Are low-temperature drying and extraction methods indicated? The best drying methods are vacuum dehydration (the most gentle) or slow, air drying (for low moisture plants). Methods such as flash-freezing damage cell structure because the expanding water bursts the cell wall. Any method involving heat can denature proteins, and destroy enzymes, vitamins, and other heat-labile factors.

Evaluating a Nutritional Supplement Company

- Does the company have an internal laboratory for testing for impurities and toxins, or does it merely rely upon letters of certification from third party suppliers.

- Does the company allow visitors to inspect its operation and facilities, or does it just put out a fancy brochure which makes them appear to be professional? Don't be fooled by companies that won't allow visitors because they are protecting some supposed trade secrets. Any company that is proud of its food supplement production wants people to come see what it does.

- Does the company conduct its own research and development or does it rely only on the research of others.

- If the company makes supplements from real foods, their facilities and methods must be inspected by the U.S. Department of Agriculture (and other government agencies). Check online for reports about the inspection results.

- Does the company conduct tests on every single batch of supplements for bacteria, fungus, pesticides, herbicides, environmental toxins (such as PCB's and mercury), rancidity, and impurities? This is a must.

Mega Quantities vs. Balanced Quantities

I could write volumes on how synthetic vitamins like thiamine castrate the descendants of the victim who uses even as much as double the daily requirement.

–Dr. Royal Lee, 1952, Lectures of Dr. Royal Lee, Vol. II[26]

Consumers are generally unaware of what supplement label data and potency claims actually mean. For instance, the most widely sold vitamin tablet in the world is vitamin C. However, according to government labeling laws, the legal definition of vitamin C is "ascorbic acid." Therefore, because only ascorbic acid may be called vitamin C, only ascorbic acid content needs to appear on label data.

However, ascorbic acid is only a single part of the whole C complex. It is to the C complex as a peel is to the banana: it protects the functional parts of the C complex from oxidation while in the growing plant. Taken alone it can provide an acidifying effect, something that can be obtained more cheaply—without creating imbalance—from apple cider vinegar.

The whole vitamin C complex, as it is structured in nature, is a combination of many substances such as organically-bound copper, bioflavonoids, and rutin. Organically-bound copper (tyrosinase) is the catalyst that activates vitamin C. Bioflavonoids and rutin are the synergists of vitamin C that keep the blood vessels and capillaries strong and prevent bruising. These factors go unmeasured in the legal definition of vitamin C.

However, because of the legal definition, manufacturers simply make a tablet with ascorbic acid and claim a high potency. This practice might be considered relatively harmless, but high dosages of ascorbic acid—an isolated chemical—can create a deficiency of its synergists. In fact, it has been repeatedly demonstrated that prolonged use of high doses of ascorbic acid, without the rest of the C complex, causes mutation and degradation of DNA within the cell, something that a natural vitamin complex could never do.[27]

---

[26] *See Appendix, AUDIO CD's section*, Lectures of Dr. Royal Lee, Vol. II

[27] *Dr. Ian Blair, Annual Meeting of the American Society for Biochemistry and Molecular Biology, June 15, 2004;* New York Times, *Jane Brody, April 09, 1998;* Nature, *Dr. Ian Podmore. April, 1998.*

Zinc is another example of how harmful it is to use mega quantities of synthetic nutrients. A deficiency of zinc will depress the immune system. Yet, too high a level of zinc, unaccompanied by the natural synergists found in food-complex zinc, will upset the balance of copper, manganese and iron, which also depresses the immune system. However, in whole foods and food-concentrate supplements, balance is always maintained, fulfilling needs without creating deficiencies.

Quality, balanced supplements[28] are possible because of a careful process developed by Dr. Royal Lee as far back as the 1930's. This process concentrates whole, chemical-free foods into supplements without breaking up nutrient complexes or destroying enzymes and synergistic factors.

Certain isolated or synthetic vitamins, such as A and D, can be toxic if taken in excess amounts. In natural food form, vitamins A and D are better processed by the body because they appear with their synergists, which help the body use and balance those nutrients.

The most significant difference between natural and synthetic vitamins is that the natural vitamin complex acts as a co-enzyme—it becomes part of the living cellular process. But the synthetic vitamin merely stimulates the body without becoming part of the cellular process. In essence then, a mega dose of a synthetic or isolated vitamin has a pharmacological effect, while a balanced food concentrate has a nutritional effect and supports physiological processes.[29] The body's rapid elimination of synthetic vitamins via the urine illustrates the temporary pharmacological action. The body treats natural vitamin complexes from food, not as waste products, but as nutrients.

---

[28] *See Appendix, About Dr. Royal Lee*
[29] *See Appendix, ARTICLES section, "Vitamin A—Toxic or Terrific?" by Judith DeCava*

CONSIDERING A NUTRITIONAL SUPPLEMENT PROGRAM

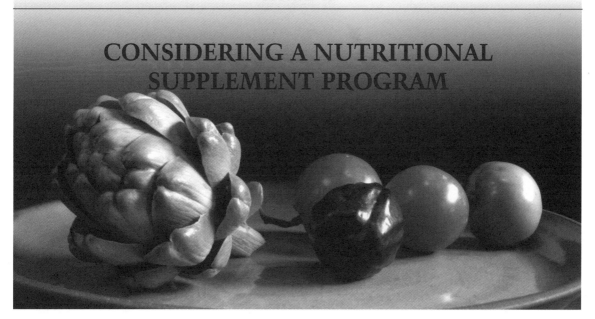

Your health professional will be recommending programs providing for your special dietary needs, supporting your return to health, and preventing illness. Diets change with the lifestyle and needs of the individual; what works nutritionally for one person may not work for another.

The dynamics to consider before recommending a food supplement program suited to any individual are *lifestyle, age, illness and injury history, symptom survey analysis, diet history, allergies and sensitivities, pregnancies, stress levels, medications, x-ray studies, handicaps, and more.*

This information, along with the analytical methods available from your health professional, will help design a nutritional program that is appropriate just for you.

Questions to Consider with Your Doctor or Health Professional

Can Nutritional Supplements Cause Nutritional Deficiencies?

It may surprise you that the answer to this question is a definite *yes*. That is why your health professional has made extensive studies of various manufacturers and their techniques in order to offer formulas made entirely from raw food rather than from heat-processed foods, or synthetic chemicals. This office makes available to you products which are whole food concentrates, containing intact enzyme systems, made from foods that are organically grown on balanced, chemical-free soil.

Scientific research has demonstrated that an excess of an isolated vitamin or mineral can produce the same symptoms as a deficiency of that vitamin or mineral. For example, high doses of isolated B vitamins can cause depletion of other B vitamins. Another example is zinc which, in excess, causes symptoms of zinc and manganese deficiency.

Balance is the key. Just as the human hand gets its dexterity from the relationship of the fingers to the thumb, a hand of all thumbs would be useless. Isolating nutrition factors from a whole complex creates imbalance, which stresses the body with toxicity and deficiency. In foods, natural forms of micronutrients are always low-dosage but high potency because of their completeness.

Are Nutritional Supplements Helpful During Pregnancy?

In every language, the first words spoken by a mother after delivery are, "Is my baby healthy?" The first words spoken by a woman upon learning she is pregnant should be, "Am I well nourished?"

The term "birth defect" refers only to structural or physiological abnormalities that develop at or before birth. However, defects in the developing fetus are most often revealed later in life. Evidence shows they often are caused by malnutrition in fetal development at a critical time when nutrients are needed to form organs. Half of all infant deaths in the US are attributed to birth defects.

Nutrition and Physical Degeneration, published in 1939 by Dr. Weston A. Price, is an enduring classic with a message that puts the people of Earth on notice: Eat right, or destroy your progeny. During the 1920s and 1930s, Dr. and Mrs. Price traveled the globe to all habitable continents photographing and recording the insidious effects of the modern diet on newly exposed indigenous people, their offspring, and their culture. Dr. Price, a superb field photographer, made a stunning visual record of the physical characteristics of native populations living on traditional diets and the subsequent altered features of their children as these family units came in contact with, and incorporated, modern adulterated foods. Irrespective of the setting—a naval base installation in the tropical South Pacific; a new trading post near the Arctic; roads built to connect previously remote alpine valleys; or encroachment of coastal cities into an arid expanse of isolated "outback" (Australia)—the result of the contact and assimilation was always the same: the indigenous people were seduced into eating what Dr. Price referred to as the "foods of commerce" (refined, processed, denatured, chemicalized non-foods). Within a single generation, their freedom from chronic disease was lost and physical degeneration set in. The next generation paid a high price, and it got worse with each subsequent generation: tooth decay, tuberculosis, physical deformities, arthritis, diabetes, diseases of the GI tract, infertility, cancer, and mental illness. Diseases, often lacking names or descriptions in the local language, soon became as common as they were in the modern "civilized" population.

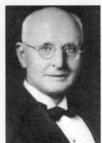
Dr. Weston A. Price.

–Excerpted from *"Prenatal Nutrition and Birth Defects"* by Mark R. Anderson[30]

Because most people today eat a diet of the "foods of commerce," nutritional supplementation with whole food concentrates is more necessary than ever for pregnant women.

---

[30] *See Appendix section, "Prenatal Nutrition and Birth Defects," by Mark R. Anderson*, Whole Food Nutrition Journal, *Volume 1 No. 2 - 2001*

Should I continue to take my other supplements after starting a supplement program at this office?

You should discuss with your health professional all the supplements you are taking to see if they can be harmoniously employed with your current program.

Iron supplements give me constipation. How can I get enough iron?

The stomach prepares iron for absorption in an acid medium. If you are taking antacids and have poor gastric secretions, you will have difficulty metabolizing iron. Most iron supplements contain an inorganic (non-food) form of iron. Very little iron is absorbed, and what remains can cause black stool and/or constipation. In a naturally-chelated food form, with proper digestion, iron is easily absorbed without causing constipation. Ask your health professional about the right form of this important blood-building mineral.

Should supplements be taken with or without food?

Good question! The answer is Yes…and No. To determine when to take a supplement depends on knowing the nature of the particular supplement and what it can achieve. Some herbs, for instance, taken on an empty stomach work differently than when taken with food. One advantage to receiving supplementation from your health professional is that he or she will know the best time to take any particular supplement.

Will there be any side effects from food supplements?

If you're taking a natural supplement, the answer is, yes—your improved health is a side effect. Furthermore, it's important to report to your health professional any reaction that occurs upon taking a supplement. This information will be invaluable in determining your ability to digest and absorb nutrients. For example, if a natural food supplement such as wheat germ oil makes you belch or feel nauseated, this is valuable feedback on the status of your gall bladder or liver. Now steps can be taken to improve your body's fat digestion rather than merely avoiding wheat germ oil, which is beneficial for healthy hair, skin and nails, and is a rich source of vitamin E complex. If you experience side effects while taking synthetic supplements, stop the supplements at once and consult your health professional about all medications, herbs and supplements you are using.

Will natural supplements interfere with any medication I'm taking?

Usually they do not. There are, however, many medications that will interfere with nutrients. And herbs have a greater propensity to interfere with medications than do nutritional supplements. Your health professional should be completely informed about all medications you are using.

Do supplements cure specific diseases?

No. Your health professional uses supplements to provide for your special dietary needs. Real food supplements give the body the fuel and protective factors it needs for proper cellular function, repair and maintenance. Supplements, like wholesome foods, support health rather than fight disease.

What about supplements for children?

The physical demands of growth can exhaust all but the best nutritional diets. Most children today are eating a chemical concoction of nutritionally empty "non-foods," the likes of which no generation in history has consumed. The inadequacies and chemical contamination of our modern food supply makes sound nutritional supplementation an important contribution to the growth and development of children.

Paying Too Little or Too Much

There is hardly anything in the
world that some man cannot make a little worse
and sell a little cheaper and
the people who consider price only
are this man's lawful prey.
It's unwise to pay too little.
When you pay too much, you
lose a little money – that is all.
When you pay too little, you sometimes lose
everything because the thing you bought was
incapable of doing
the thing it was bought to do.
The common law of business balance
prohibits paying a little and getting a lot —
it cannot be done.
If you deal with the lowest bidder, it is well to add
something for the risk you run. And if you do
that, you will have enough to pay for something
better.

- John Ruskin,
19th Century English Philosopher

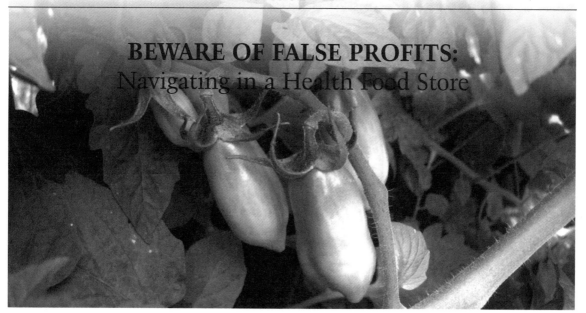

BEWARE OF FALSE PROFITS:
Navigating in a Health Food Store

There probably hasn't been a civilization in recorded history that did not have dietary beliefs about food and health. But, to our knowledge, the health food store is a phenomenon unique to this current civilization and time. Apothecaries, herbal, medicinal and healing shops have occupied their place in business over the centuries, but a shop dedicated to selling "whole" foods, or "organic," "natural," "fresh," or "alternative" foods is evidence that we are split between an awareness of what healthy food is and is not.

Unfortunately, the original vision of health food stores supplying honestly whole, fresh, organic, unadulterated foods came and went with the sixties. What we have instead are new ways of marketing food that is still conventional and almost as adulterated as the common supermarket brands, peppered with some organic produce, grains, nuts, higher quality oils and, in some cases, healthier meats.

Bakery goods and deli foods are very often made with white sugar and white flour and preservatives—in health food stores! Quality whole food does not need sugar or chemicals for flavor. Sugar and chemicals are not "whole food." Yet, health food stores promote and sell more non-healthy food than health food. The reason: This is business not health. This is what sells, not what nourishes. Clever marketing has enabled health food stores to pass off mediocre food as health food—about as original as snake oil, but it works.

The free-market is a great place for people to express creative ideas, make money, and contribute the gift of their unique dreams to society. But so-called health food stores are raking in the profits based on a *pretense* of healthy products. Yet, regulation of business, in a futile attempt to police the integrity of business owners, is not the solution—nor should it be. Such regulation has an antibiotic effect (anti-life); it oppresses the creativity and freedom of those who *do* have integrity. Instead, let's develop an informed public who knows where to spend their money in order to nurture and protect their health. This alone weeds out the snake oil salesmen.

Health food store history is littered with pioneering health food stores and companies whose rugged independence was stifled by the huge conventional health food companies; they either had to close shop or sell themselves to the larger store. Again, that's life in the free market. But the dominating companies do a great disservice by promoting cheaper products, sold at a premium, rather than expanding the market for real food. This approach is in contrast to the impetus behind the creation of health food stores which was to cultivate a **real foods** market by educating about, and providing, real food products. Good examples of promoting cheaper products are: the predominance of conventional produce over organic in most health food stores (where there should not be ANY commercial, pesticide/herbicide laden produce) and **ultra**-pasteurized dairy products. If health food stores had cultivated the raw dairy market, consumer demand could have caused raw dairy products to be legal today; children would be growing up with one of Nature's highest quality foods available to them on a daily basis.

If you shop in any health food store, read labels, ask questions, write feedback in comment boxes, and call executives to tell them you want honest health food. But you will profit far more from dedicating time and energy to finding truly honest local farmers, Community Supported Agriculture farms and dairies, farm stands, shops and websites that sell real food. You can prepare simple, healthy meals out of real foods that, in the long run, save you time and money. *Think suffering, medical bills and sick days.*

Another misuse of health food stores is asking for health advice. Health food employees are not health practitioners and cannot be relied upon for medical or health information. It's difficult enough for the professional to learn all there is to know about the latest research and findings, as well as have the experience necessary to help others. It will be far more safe and intelligent to find an informed doctor or health practitioner to guide you.

Counterfeit vs. Original Food

Original foods are the basic meat, fish, legumes, seeds, nuts, vegetables, fruits, grains, and dairy products out of which nutrient-rich meals are made. **Counterfeit foods** are food products that (1) look like original foods but have been grown on depleted soil and treated with chemicals, (2) are processed into packaged or fast-food forms, resulting in significant loss of nutrients and enzymes, (3) contain unfit ingredients such as altered fats, as well as chemicals, hormones, artificial flavors, refined and artificial sugars, etc.

Can you tell the difference between counterfeit and original food when shopping in any market, including a health food store? Here's a handy tool to help you find a genuine health food store:

Healthy Health Food Store Checklist

✔ They stock only organic food instead of **any** conventional food. *After all, you could go to your local supermarket and buy the same conventional produce **at lower prices**.*

✔ They don't sell farm-raised fish (aqua farming), only wild fish. *Aqua-farmed fish are raised on antibiotics and non-organic fish chow.*

✔ They do not promote aisles filled to the brim with junk, sugary, or snack foods, such as corn-syrup-laden soda, fried chips, and cookies (made with cheap ingredients such as hydrogenated oils and refined sugars), offering inferior nutrition and abundant calories. *This is one of the food frauds that drove people from conventional markets in the first place.*

✔ They do not sell pasteurized juices. *Pasteurized juice offers nothing but carbohydrates (sugar) because all nutrients and enzymes are destroyed by pasteurization.*

✔ They do not sell deli foods laced with sugar-sweetened sauces. *If we wanted to eat dessert for lunch, we'd dine in the bakery.*

✔ They do not entice you with baked goods made from perished, enriched, refined wheat flour. *Remember, flour is as perishable as a freshly cut apple; the oils in perished flour are rancid from oxygenation.*

✔ They do not stock aisles full of synthetic vitamins as well as various supplements of dubious quality. *This would be antithetical to the seminal idea of a health food store for reasons already fully covered previously in this book.*

✔ They don't sell processed, packaged cereals fortified with artificial vitamins. *After all, you can buy those in a conventional supermarket **at lower prices.** Conventional cereals might not contain organically-raised grains, but even organically raised grains, once processed into dry cereal, have little nutrient value.*

✔ They don't sell any product, including toothpaste, containing fluoride. *Adding a non-nutritive, toxic chemical to an otherwise natural product… is so blatantly unprincipled that it makes my hair hurt!*

✔ They don't sell any food or dessert made with refined, white sugar or hydrogenated oil, or oils unfit for human consumption. They don't sell pasteurized or ultra-pasteurized milk, or pasteurized honey or refined maple syrup. They do not sell mayonnaise made from inferior ingredients such as canola oil and sweeteners. The man or woman at the meat counter does not shrug impatiently and tell you that they have to put sugar in the pork sausage because it preserves the meat without using nitrates or nitrites. Instead, he or she will smile proudly and tell you that people have been drying and curing and preserving meat and fish for thousands of years without either sugar or preservatives. He or she will go on to inform you of the hyper-destructive effect on proteins when they are cooked with sugar. He will remind you of the exact, precise reason the idea of health food stores dawned on us in the first place: To provide whole, unadulterated food to the general public as an alternative to broken and adulterated food. *Seems to us this is still a great concept just waiting for a few energetic, dedicated entrepreneurs to bring into reality.*

So carry your checklist with you and see if you can find a **real** health food store. And please call us toll-free if you do. In fact, call us toll-free if you even find raw, organic wheat germ that is nitrogen-packed to prevent rancidity. We will surely reward you.

By the way, we thank and congratulate any real health food stores out there for sticking to their principles. Let us know who you are and we will tell the world about you.

Meanwhile, don't be fooled by sheep in wolves' clothing. The modern health food store can be a dangerous terrain to navigate.

If we teach children at a young age that by their eating habits they will determine the health of the next generation, they will learn responsibility in all areas of life. It might even be said that the lack of a sense of responsibility that characterizes so much of modern government and industry today is an outgrowth of the attitude that the way we eat has no bearing on the health of our children and grandchildren.

–Sally Fallon

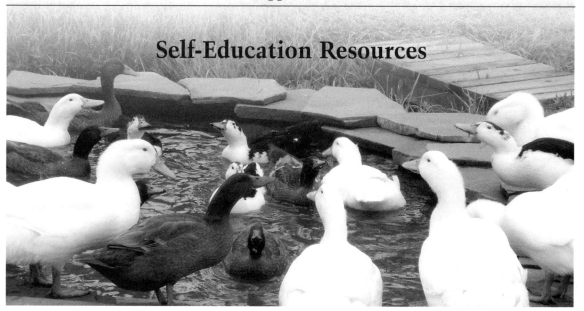

Self-Education Resources

Educational information about health and how to properly care for our bodies and the soil is abundantly available through many sources. Don't be fooled into waiting for dramatic breakthroughs promised in the popular press. More than enough is already known today to ensure a strong, healthy life. Only a fraction of this knowledge is generally reported and implemented. Fortunately, the internet and freedom of the press makes materials for self-education highly accessible.

In fact, the challenge now is sorting through all the information and knowing what is sound and what is not. Discerning what is best for your present needs will become easier as you develop a wholesome lifestyle. Professional assistance is crucial and can prove to be your most valuable resource for information and guidance. Seek the advice of your health professional for information on how to accomplish your goals and where to find more knowledge and wisdom on nutrition and health.

We Highly Recommend the Following Materials for Further Self-Education in the Topics Considered in this Book

Books

A Hunza Trip: The Wheel of Health, by Dr. Bernard Jensen and G. T. Wrench, M.D. See all books by Bernard Jensen, PhD, DC, published by Bernard Jensen International, **www.bernardjensen.org**

Nourishing Traditions, The Cookbook that Challenges Politically Correct Nutrition and the Diet Dictocrats, by Sally Fallon, with Mary G. Enig, call New Trends Publishing, **877-707-1776**, **www.newtrendspublishing.com**, or Selene River Press, **866-407-9323**, **www.seleneriverpress.com**

Know Your Fats: The Complete Primer for Understanding the Nutrition of Fats, Oils and Cholesterol, by Mary G. Enig, the first person to speak out about the dangers of trans fatty acids in the food supply in spite of industry blackballing. Available from booksellers and Selene River Press, 866-407-9323, **www.seleneriverpress.com**

Sugar Blues, by William Dufty, published by Chilton Books, Radnor, PA, Selene River Press, **866-407-9323, www.seleneriverpress.com,** and booksellers.

Empty Harvest, the Link Between the Soil and Our Immune System, by Dr. Bernard Jensen and Mark R. Anderson, from Selene River Press, **866-407-9323, www.seleneriverpress.com,** and booksellers.

Lectures of Dr. Royal Lee, Volume I and II, compiled by Mark R. Anderson, [Volume II is a 32-CD box set; go to **AUDIO CD's**], are available only through Selene River Press, **866-407-9323, www.seleneriverpress.com**

Nutrition and Physical Degeneration, by Dr. Weston Price, available from The Price-Pottenger Foundation, **800-366-3748, www.pricepottinger.org,** and Selene River Press, **866-407-9323, www.seleneriverpress.com**

The Real Truth about Vitamins and Anti-Oxidants (and all other books) by Judith DeCava, MS, LNC, Selene River Press, **866-407-9323, www.seleneriverpress.com**

Food Fundamentals (and all other books) by Judith DeCava, MS, LNC, Selene River Press, **866-407-9323, www.seleneriverpress.com**

Handbook to Health, with Menus and Recipes by Vivian Rice and Edie Wogaman, Selene River Press, 866-407-9323, **www.seleneriverpress.com**

Don't Drink Your Milk! New Frightening Medical Facts About the World's Most Overrated Nutrient, by Frank A. Oski, M.D., all booksellers.

The Untold Story of Milk, by Ron Schmid, N.D., available on **www.amazon.com**

Pottenger's Cats, A Study in Nutrition, by Francis M. Pottenger, M.D., Selene River Press, **866-407-9323, www.seleneriverpress.com,** and booksellers.

Studies in Deficiency Disease, by Sir Major General William McCarrison, M.D. available as a free downloadable Acrobat file from the Selene River Press website, "Historical Archives" Section, **www.seleneriverpress.com**

New Trends Publishing, Important Books on Diet and Health (includes Sally Fallon's books), **877-707-1776, www.newtrendspublishing.com**

"Acres USA, A Voice for Eco-Agriculture," 800-355-5313, www.acresusa.com

"News and Views...on Nutritional Therapeutics," Vol.1-8, 1997-2004, CD compilation of Judith DeCava's newsletter for health professionals, only from Selene River Press, 866-407-9323, www.seleneriverpress.com

"Wild Rice, A Holistic Newsletter," by Vivian Rice and Marjorie Carroll, published monthly. Their recipes, health tips, short useful articles and Vivian's irrepressible humor are a welcome read every time. Call for info: 719-635-5596.

"Wise Traditions, in Food, Farming and the Healing Arts," is a publication of The Weston A. Price Foundation, edited by Sally Fallon, (202) 333-HEAL (4325), www.WestonAPrice.org

Articles

WATER

"Ideal Drinking Water," by Dr. Royal Lee, D.D.S., *Let's Live Magazine*, available free from the Historical Archives at Selene River Press, 866-407-9323, www.seleneriverpress.com

FOOD

"Food Fights, Part I and II," by Judith DeCava, C.C.N, L.N.C., article in newsletter, Nutrition News and Views...on Nutritional Therapeutics, Vol.5 No.3, available on CD-ROM from 866-407-9323, www.seleneriverpress.com

PREGNANCY

"Prenatal Nutrition and Birth Defects," by Mark R. Anderson, published in Whole Food Nutrition Journal, Volume 1 No. 2 – 2001, available free from the Historical Archives at Selene River Press, 866-407-9323, www.seleneriverpress.com

VITAMIN A

"Vitamin A—Toxic or Terrific," by Judith DeCava, Nutrition News and Views...on Nutritional Therapeutics, July/August 2004, available through newsletter subscription or your area Standard Process Representative or Distributor, who can be found at www.standardprocess.com. Contact Selene River Press for future CD-ROM collections of this newsletter.

Lectures of Dr. Royal Lee, Volume II, compiled by Mark R. Anderson, [**NOTE:** Volume I is a book; go to **BOOKS**], available only through Selene River Press, **866-407-9323**, **www.seleneriverpress.com**

Resources

SELENE RIVER PRESS, INC., Publisher and Distributor of Select Books on Health, provides a free CD-Rom Catalog; *The Selene River Press Collection, A Catalog of Self-Health Literacy,* and is dedicated to the publication and distribution of books, tools, and resources that support and guide lifelong learning in the art and science of health through nutrition. Call for a free CD-catalog, or download it from their website, to order many of the materials listed here for self-education. **866-407-9323, 970-407-9323, www.seleneriverpress.com**

FREE HEALTH E-NEWSLETTER: "**eHealthy News You Can Use,**" Dr. Joseph Mercola publishes articles from a wide variety of sources about health, recommends products and books, and has a good search service. **www.mercola.com**

LISTING OF HEALTHY MEAT AND FOOD: Shopping Guide 2004, for Finding the Healthiest Foods in the Supermarkets and Health Food Stores, by Sally Fallon, is a handy pamphlet listing brands and contact information for many of the higher quality foods on the market, available from The Weston A. Price Foundation, **202-333-HEAL (4325)** (See below)

Foundations

THE WESTON A. PRICE FOUNDATION, in their own words,

> *The Foundation is dedicated to restoring nutrient-dense foods to the human diet through education, research and activism. It supports a number of movements that contribute to this objective including accurate nutrition instruction, organic and biodynamic farming, pasture-feeding of livestock, community-supported farms, honest and informative labeling, prepared parenting and nurturing therapies. Specific goals include establishment of universal access to clean, certified raw milk and a ban on the use of soy formula for infants.*

202-333-HEAL (4325), www.WestonAPrice.org, WestonAPrice@msn.com

REAL MILK, founded by Sally Fallon, is a campaign for real milk and a project of the Weston A. Price Foundation. "Back in the '20s, Americans could buy fresh raw whole milk, real clabber and buttermilk, luscious naturally yellow butter, fresh farm cheeses and cream in various colors and thicknesses. Today's milk is accused of causing everything from allergies to heart disease to cancer, but when Americans could buy Real Milk, these diseases were rare. In fact, a supply of high quality dairy products was considered vital to American security and the economic well being of the nation. What's needed today is a return to humane, non-toxic, pasture-based dairying and small-scale traditional processing, in short…a campaign for real milk."

www.realmilk.com, **www.WestonAPrice.org**

THE PRICE-POTTENGER FOUNDATION, in their own words,

Through the dissemination of the ancestral wisdom practiced by pre-industrial societies, and through modern scientific validation of the principles of sound nutrition, the Price-Pottenger Nutrition Foundation (PPNF) provides guidance for the reversal of modern "civilized" dietary trends that promote disease and physical & mental degeneration.

The Foundation is dedicated to achieving the optimum expression of our human genetic potential and harmony with nature's laws through the right use of technology and the practical application of the principles of sound nutrition. PPNF provides accurate information on whole foods and proper preparation techniques, soil improvement, natural farming, pure water, non-toxic dentistry and holistic therapies in order to conquer disease; prevent birth defects; avoid personality disturbances & delinquency; enhance the environment; and enable all people to achieve long life and excellent health, now and into the 21st century.

To assure the healing professionals and the public would always have access to the critical nutritional discoveries of Dr. Price, the Foundation has a mandate to maintain in print his Nutrition and Physical Degeneration as it contains the documentation of his research.

800-366-3748, **www.price-pottenger.org**

Community Supported Agriculture And Real Milk

GUIDESTONE CSA GARDEN AND DAIRY: David Lynch, the agricultural director, is nationally recognized as an inspirational speaker for the sustainable agriculture movement. He was a founding member of The Stewardship Community in 1988 and helped start COPA (Colorado Organic Producers Association). The Stewardship community is an environmental education organization that demonstrates and teaches sustainable living skills. They have sponsored many conferences and workshops around the topic of sustainable farming and earth stewardship. They run their farm as a Community Supported Agriculture model, producing organic cow milk, meat, vegetables, eggs, honey, and wood fired stone-oven breads. They also provide up to 12-month internships for those committed to learning how to create a financially sustainable demonstration farm around sustainable agriculture and the CSA model. **970-461-0771, www.stewardshipcommunity.org, www.guidestonefarm.com**

PURIFICATION AND INFORMATION

Aqua MD, **www.aquamd.com**

Ozark Water Service and Environmental Services: Warren Clough, Analytical Chemist and Water Consultant. **800-835-8908, 501-298-3421**

LOCAL WATER SERVICES

Check with your city for a copy of the "Consumer Confidence Report." Cities are required by law to make this report available about the contents of their water. All water testing they do is public record, for the asking, so call to find out what is available to you.

FLUORIDE

Empty Harvest, by Dr. Bernard Jensen and Mark R. Anderson, *Food Fundamentals* and *Conquering Cancer*, by Judith DeCava. See **BOOKS** section.

Fluoride Action Network is an international coalition working to end water fluoridation and alert the public to fluoride's health and environmental risks. **802-355-0999 www.flouridealert.org**

BREAD

Natural Bridge Bakery, bread made in the Old World Flemish tradition of desem baking. Desem (pronounced day'-zum) is the starter that leavens the dough using the micro-organisms that occur naturally on the grain itself. Through slow fermentation, they produce highly digestible bread. Organic grain is freshly milled for each Natural Bridge bake, using a stone-burr grist mill. This keeps the flour cool, preserving its nutrients. After two days of careful preparation, Natural Bridge loaves are baked in a massive wood-fired brick oven. With its low dome and deep chamber, this oven yields full-flavored, chewy, crusty, fine-textured bread. Order from The Grain and Salt Society, **800-867-7258, www.celtic-seasalt.com**

COD LIVER OIL

Blue Ice Pure Cod Liver Oil, unique cod liver oil produced in Norway. The cod is seasonally fished and exclusively harvested from the icy blue Artic Ocean, and the oil is molecularly distilled, all to ensure a premium quality, naturally high-vitamin Cod Liver Oil. Green Pastures, **402-338-5551 www.greenpasture.org (NOTE: The web address is "pasture" *not* "pastures.")**

HONEY

Really Raw Honey, 800-732-5729, **www.reallyrawhoney.com**

Sweet William of Earlville, 315-691-6600, **www.rawhoney.com**
Dan McLaughlin, for small quantities when available call 970-663-0848, or write Dan at 6501 Chipper Lane, Loveland, Colorado 80537.

Hawaiian White Honey, available at Whole Foods Market, Republic of Tea **www.republicoftea.com** and easily found by searching on the web.

MILK

Organic Pastures, Blaine and Mark McAfee, produce certified Grade A, pasture-grazed raw milk, and ship right to your door their delicious, healthy products: raw milk, cream, colostrum milk, butter, buttermilk and more. Call to order: **877-RawMilk (729-6455)**, **www.organicpastures.com**

SEA SALT

The Grain & Salt Society carries high quality Celtic sea salt, olives, breads and other goodies. **800-867-7258, www.celtic-seasalt.com**

Flour Mills

Both of the following recommendations are home flour mills using the natural stone, carborundum, which is second only to diamonds in hardness, so it never needs replacing. There is no loss of nutrient factors because both mills grind without overheating the grain. You can check into each to compare which one might be best for you.

LEE HOUSEHOLD FLOUR MILL, comes in four models. The design is a Dr. Royal Lee original being made today by EM Lee Engineering in Milwaukee, WI, **414-272-4050**

GRANO 200 ELECTRIC STONE MILL BY SCHNITZER, can be ordered from Juicers for Less, **888-392-9237, www.juicersforless.com**

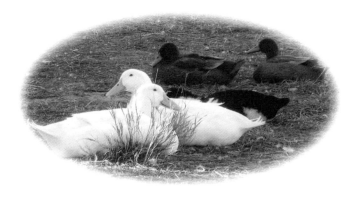

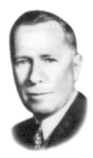

Dr. Royal Lee

Dr. Royal Lee founded Vitamin Products Company in 1929, a whole food supplement company which he eventually renamed Standard Process Laboratories.

Raised on a farm his Norwegian grandfather settled in 1845 near Dodgeville, Wisconsin, the young Lee's interest in science and nutrition began early at the local elementary school. At age 12, he compiled a notebook of definitions on biochemistry and nutrition, and he began collecting books on these subjects. A collection that started as a hobby continued throughout his lifetime to eventually become part of the Dr. Royal Lee Memorial Library.

After serving in the First World War, Dr. Lee graduated in 1924 from Marquette University Dental School in Wisconsin. While attending the university, his primary interest became the importance of nutrition. A paper he prepared in 1923 outlined the relationship of vitamin deficiency to tooth decay and showed the necessity of vitamins in the diet. His research led to the development of CATALYN®, a vitamin concentrate derived from whole foods. Introduced in 1929, CATALYN became the nucleus of a complete line of nutritional supplements at the Vitamin Products Company.

Dr. Lee believed the key to maintaining the quality of nutritional supplements was a unique manufacturing process. He designed high-vacuum, low-temperature drying equipment to preserve the living enzyme systems of the whole foods. These technologies continue to be used today. From a small two-room facility, the Vitamin Products Company has evolved into the present company we call Standard Process, Inc., in Palmyra, Wisconsin. Standard Process is still family-owned and operated. Their large certified organic farms serve as a source for most of the whole food supplements they manufacture, as well as a model for agricultural groups and organizations interested in learning large-scale organic farming methods. The company is continually growing, building on expert research and quality manufacturing first imposed by Dr. Lee.

In addition to his work in the nutrition field, Dr. Lee was the inventor of a wide variety of dental, mechanical, automotive and electrical equipment. He filed over 70 patents for all types of equipment, processes, internal combustion engines and food products. For more information on Dr. Lee and Standard Process products, call **800-848-5061**, or visit their website at **www.standardprocess.com**